Table Of Contents

Chapter 1: Understanding Probiotics

The Role of Probiotics in Gut Health

Probiotics play a crucial role in maintaining optimal gut health for women over 30. These live bacteria and yeasts are known to promote a healthy balance of gut flora, which is essential for proper digestion and overall wellness. Probiotics can help improve gut health by replenishing beneficial bacteria in the gut, reducing inflammation, and promoting hormonal balance.

One of the key benefits of probiotics for gut health is their ability to support weight management. Research has shown that a healthy gut microbiome is linked to a lower risk of obesity and weight gain. Probiotics can help regulate appetite, reduce cravings for unhealthy foods, and improve metabolism, making it easier for women over 30 to maintain a healthy weight.

In addition to their role in weight management, probiotics can also improve digestion by enhancing nutrient absorption and reducing symptoms of bloating, gas, and constipation. By supporting a healthy balance of gut bacteria, probiotics can help women over 30 experience better digestion and overall gut health.

Furthermore, probiotics have been shown to reduce inflammation in the gut, which is linked to a variety of health issues, including autoimmune diseases, allergies, and skin conditions. By promoting a healthy gut microbiome, probiotics can help reduce inflammation and improve overall immune function in women over 30.

Finally, probiotics can also play a role in hormonal balance for women over 30. The gut microbiome is intricately connected to hormone production and regulation, and probiotics can help support a healthy balance of hormones. By promoting gut health through the use of probiotics, women over 30 can experience improved hormonal balance and overall wellness.

Benefits of Probiotics for Women Over 30

As women age, maintaining good gut health becomes increasingly important for overall well-being. Probiotics are live bacteria and yeasts that are beneficial for digestive health, and they can offer a wide range of benefits for women over 30. In this subchapter, we will explore the specific advantages of incorporating probiotics into your daily routine.

One of the key benefits of probiotics for women over 30 is improved gut health. As we age, our digestive systems can become less efficient, leading to issues like bloating, gas, and constipation. Probiotics help to restore the balance of good bacteria in the gut, promoting smoother digestion and reducing these uncomfortable symptoms. By supporting a healthy gut microbiome, probiotics can also boost energy levels and immune function.

In addition to aiding digestion, probiotics can also play a role in weight management for women over 30. Research has shown that certain strains of probiotics can help to regulate appetite, reduce fat storage, and even increase metabolism. By incorporating probiotic-rich foods or supplements into your diet, you may find it easier to maintain a healthy weight and support your overall wellness goals.

Furthermore, probiotics have been shown to have anti-inflammatory properties, which can be particularly beneficial for women over 30. Chronic inflammation is linked to a range of health issues, including heart disease, diabetes, and autoimmune disorders. By reducing inflammation in the gut, probiotics can help to protect against these conditions and support long-term health.

Another important benefit of probiotics for women over 30 is their impact on hormonal balance. The gut microbiome plays a crucial role in producing and metabolizing hormones, and imbalances in gut bacteria can contribute to hormonal issues like PMS, menopause symptoms, and thyroid dysfunction. By supporting a healthy gut with probiotics, women can help to regulate their hormones and improve their overall well-being.

Overall, incorporating probiotics into your daily routine can offer a wide range of benefits for women over 30, including improved gut health, weight management, reduced inflammation, and hormonal balance. By prioritizing your digestive wellness and taking steps to support a healthy gut microbiome, you can promote better overall health and vitality as you age.

Chapter 2: Gut Health and Weight Management

How Gut Health Affects Weight

Our gut health plays a crucial role in maintaining a healthy weight, especially for women over 30. The balance of good and bad bacteria in our gut can impact our metabolism, digestion, and even our hormonal balance. Probiotics, which are live beneficial bacteria, can help improve gut health and support weight management.

When the balance of bacteria in our gut is disrupted, it can lead to weight gain and difficulty losing weight. Studies have shown that a healthy gut microbiome is essential for maintaining a healthy weight. Probiotics can help restore this balance by promoting the growth of beneficial bacteria and reducing the harmful effects of bad bacteria.

In addition to supporting weight management, a healthy gut can also improve digestion. When our gut is functioning properly, we can better absorb nutrients from the foods we eat, which can help us feel more satisfied and reduce cravings. Probiotics can help improve digestion by aiding in the breakdown of food and promoting the absorption of essential nutrients.

Furthermore, a healthy gut can help reduce inflammation in the body, which is linked to weight gain and chronic diseases. Probiotics have been shown to have anti-inflammatory effects, which can help reduce inflammation in the gut and throughout the body. By reducing inflammation, we can support weight management and improve overall health.

Lastly, our gut health is closely connected to our hormonal balance. The gut produces and regulates hormones that can impact our appetite, metabolism, and even our mood. Probiotics can help support hormonal balance by promoting the production of beneficial hormones and reducing the levels of harmful hormones. By improving gut health, we can support weight management and maintain overall well-being as women over 30.

Using Probiotics to Support Weight Management

Probiotics have gained popularity in recent years for their ability to support gut health. But did you know that these beneficial bacteria can also play a role in weight management? For women over 30 looking to maintain a healthy weight, incorporating probiotics into their daily routine can be a game-changer. Not only do probiotics help improve digestion and reduce inflammation in the gut, but they can also help regulate hormonal balance, which is essential for maintaining a healthy weight.

When it comes to weight management, gut health is key. Research has shown that the balance of bacteria in the gut can have a significant impact on weight. Probiotics help promote the growth of beneficial bacteria in the gut, which can help improve digestion and absorption of nutrients. This can lead to better weight management and overall health. By incorporating probiotics into your daily routine, you can support a healthy gut and in turn, support your weight management goals.

One of the ways that probiotics support weight management is by reducing inflammation in the gut. Chronic inflammation in the gut can lead to weight gain and other health issues. Probiotics help reduce inflammation by promoting a healthy balance of bacteria in the gut, which can help improve digestion and prevent inflammation. By incorporating probiotics into your daily routine, you can support a healthy gut and reduce inflammation, which can help support weight management.

In addition to improving digestion and reducing inflammation, probiotics can also help regulate hormonal balance, which is essential for maintaining a healthy weight. Hormonal imbalances can lead to weight gain and other health issues. Probiotics help support hormonal balance by promoting a healthy balance of bacteria in the

gut, which can help regulate hormones related to weight
management. By incorporating probiotics into your daily routine,
you can support a healthy gut and hormonal balance, which can help
support weight management.

In conclusion, probiotics can play a significant role in supporting
weight management for women over 30. By improving digestion,
reducing inflammation, and regulating hormonal balance, probiotics
can help support a healthy gut and in turn, support weight
management goals. Incorporating probiotics into your daily routine
can be a simple and effective way to support your overall health and
well-being.

Chapter 3: Gut Health and Digestion

Common Digestive Issues in Women Over 30

As women age, their digestive systems can become more susceptible to various issues that can impact their overall health and well-being. In particular, women over 30 may experience common digestive issues that can be both uncomfortable and debilitating if left untreated. In this subchapter, we will explore some of the most prevalent digestive issues that affect women over 30 and how probiotics can play a crucial role in maintaining gut health.

One of the most common digestive issues that women over 30 may face is irritable bowel syndrome (IBS). IBS can cause symptoms such as bloating, gas, diarrhea, and abdominal pain, making it challenging to go about daily life comfortably. Probiotics have been shown to help alleviate symptoms of IBS by restoring balance to the gut microbiome and reducing inflammation in the digestive tract.

Another common digestive issue that women over 30 may encounter is acid reflux, also known as gastroesophageal reflux disease (GERD). Acid reflux occurs when stomach acid flows back into the esophagus, causing a burning sensation in the chest and throat. Probiotics can help regulate stomach acid levels and improve digestion, potentially reducing the frequency and severity of acid reflux episodes.

Women over 30 may also experience changes in their gut health that can impact their weight management efforts. Imbalances in the gut microbiome can lead to weight gain and difficulty losing weight, even with a healthy diet and regular exercise. Probiotics can help support a healthy metabolism and promote weight loss by improving digestion and nutrient absorption.

In addition to digestive issues, women over 30 may also be at risk for inflammation in the gut, which can contribute to a variety of health conditions, including autoimmune diseases and chronic pain. Probiotics can help reduce inflammation in the gut by promoting the growth of beneficial bacteria and strengthening the intestinal barrier, which can prevent harmful substances from entering the bloodstream and triggering an immune response.

Finally, hormonal imbalances can also impact gut health in women over 30, leading to symptoms such as bloating, mood swings, and irregular bowel movements. Probiotics can help regulate hormone levels by supporting the production of neurotransmitters in the gut and balancing estrogen and progesterone levels. By incorporating probiotics into their daily routine, women over 30 can improve their digestive health and overall well-being.

Improving Digestive Health with Probiotics

Probiotics have gained popularity in recent years for their ability to improve digestive health. For women over 30, maintaining a healthy gut is essential for overall wellness. Probiotics are live bacteria and yeasts that are good for your health, especially your digestive system. These "good" bacteria can help keep your gut healthy by restoring the natural balance of bacteria in your gut, which can be disrupted by factors such as stress, diet, and aging.

One key benefit of probiotics for women over 30 is their ability to aid in weight management. Studies have shown that certain strains of probiotics can help with weight loss and prevent weight gain. By promoting a healthy balance of gut bacteria, probiotics can help regulate metabolism and reduce inflammation in the body, leading to better weight management outcomes.

In addition to weight management, probiotics can also improve digestion for women over 30. As we age, our digestive system may become less efficient, leading to issues such as bloating, gas, and constipation. Probiotics can help by promoting the growth of beneficial bacteria in the gut, which can aid in the breakdown of food and absorption of nutrients. This can lead to better digestion and overall gut health.

Furthermore, probiotics have been shown to reduce inflammation in the gut, which can help with a variety of digestive issues such as irritable bowel syndrome (IBS) and inflammatory bowel disease (IBD). By promoting a healthy balance of gut bacteria, probiotics can help reduce inflammation and promote healing in the gut, leading to improved digestive health and overall wellness for women over 30.

Lastly, probiotics can also play a role in balancing hormones for women over 30. The gut is often referred to as the "second brain" due to its connection to the central nervous system and its influence on hormone production. By promoting a healthy balance of gut bacteria, probiotics can help regulate hormone levels, leading to improved hormonal balance and overall well-being for women over 30. Incorporating probiotics into your daily routine can have a significant impact on your digestive health and overall wellness as you age.

Chapter 4: Gut Health and Inflammation

Understanding Inflammation in the Gut

Inflammation in the gut is a common issue that many women over 30 face, and it can have a significant impact on digestive wellness. Understanding what causes inflammation in the gut is crucial in order to effectively manage and improve gut health. In this subchapter, we will delve into the various factors that contribute to gut inflammation and how probiotics can play a key role in alleviating inflammation and promoting overall digestive wellness.

One of the main causes of gut inflammation is an imbalance of bacteria in the gut. When harmful bacteria outnumber beneficial bacteria, it can lead to inflammation and various digestive issues. Probiotics are live bacteria and yeasts that are beneficial for gut health, as they help restore the balance of good bacteria in the gut. By incorporating probiotics into your daily routine, you can reduce inflammation in the gut and promote a healthy digestive system.

Another factor that can contribute to gut inflammation is poor dietary choices. Processed foods, high in sugar and unhealthy fats, can trigger inflammation in the gut and disrupt the delicate balance of bacteria. By consuming a diet rich in whole foods, high in fiber, and low in processed foods, you can reduce inflammation in the gut and support a healthy microbiome. Probiotic-rich foods such as yogurt, kefir, sauerkraut, and kombucha are excellent choices for promoting gut health and reducing inflammation.

Stress is also a major contributor to gut inflammation. Chronic stress can disrupt the gut-brain axis, leading to inflammation and digestive issues. By practicing stress-reducing techniques such as meditation, yoga, deep breathing exercises, and getting plenty of rest, you can lower inflammation in the gut and improve overall digestive wellness. Probiotics have also been shown to have a positive impact on stress levels, as they can help regulate the production of neurotransmitters that influence mood and stress.

Inflammation in the gut can also affect hormonal balance in women over 30. The gut plays a crucial role in hormone regulation, as it is responsible for metabolizing hormones and eliminating excess estrogen from the body. When inflammation disrupts the gut microbiome, it can lead to hormonal imbalances and a host of health issues. By supporting gut health with probiotics, you can reduce inflammation in the gut, promote hormonal balance, and improve overall well-being. In the following chapters, we will explore how probiotics can aid in weight management, digestion, and hormonal balance, and provide practical tips for incorporating probiotics into your daily routine for optimal gut health.

Using Probiotics to Reduce Inflammation

In recent years, the use of probiotics to reduce inflammation in the body has gained significant attention, especially among women over 30 who are looking to improve their gut health. Probiotics are live bacteria and yeasts that are beneficial for the digestive system. These good bacteria can help restore balance in the gut microbiome, which plays a crucial role in maintaining overall health.

One of the key benefits of using probiotics to reduce inflammation is their ability to support the immune system. Research has shown that a healthy gut microbiome can help regulate the body's inflammatory response, reducing the risk of chronic inflammation-related conditions such as autoimmune diseases, allergies, and even cancer. By consuming probiotic-rich foods or supplements, women can help support their immune system and reduce inflammation in the body.

Furthermore, probiotics have been shown to have a positive impact on gut health and weight management. Studies have found that certain strains of probiotics can help regulate appetite, improve metabolism, and even reduce fat storage in the body. By incorporating probiotic-rich foods like yogurt, kefir, sauerkraut, and kimchi into their diet, women over 30 can support their weight management goals while also reducing inflammation in the body.

In addition to supporting weight management, probiotics can also play a key role in promoting healthy digestion. By maintaining a balanced gut microbiome, probiotics can help improve digestion, reduce bloating, and alleviate symptoms of conditions like Irritable Bowel Syndrome (IBS) and constipation. This can lead to overall better gut health and increased comfort for women dealing with digestive issues.

Overall, incorporating probiotics into your daily routine can have a profound impact on reducing inflammation in the body, promoting gut health, supporting weight management, improving digestion, and even balancing hormonal levels. As women over 30, it is essential to prioritize our gut health and overall well-being, and probiotics can be a valuable tool in achieving optimal health and vitality. By making small changes to our diet and lifestyle, we can harness the power of probiotics to reduce inflammation and improve our quality of life.

Chapter 5: Gut Health and Hormonal Balance

The Gut-Hormone Connection

In recent years, there has been a growing body of research demonstrating the intricate connection between our gut health and our hormones. This connection, known as the gut-hormone connection, plays a crucial role in maintaining overall health and well-being, particularly for women over 30. Understanding how our gut health impacts our hormonal balance can empower us to take control of our health and make informed choices to support our bodies.

One of the key players in the gut-hormone connection is the microbiome, the community of trillions of bacteria that reside in our gut. These bacteria play a vital role in regulating our hormones, including estrogen and cortisol, by producing and metabolizing hormones. When the balance of these bacteria is disrupted, it can lead to hormonal imbalances and a host of health issues, from weight gain to mood swings.

Probiotics, the beneficial bacteria found in fermented foods and supplements, can help support a healthy gut microbiome and promote hormonal balance. By introducing probiotics into our diet, we can help restore the balance of bacteria in our gut, which in turn can have a positive impact on our hormonal health. Studies have shown that certain strains of probiotics can help regulate estrogen levels, reduce cortisol production, and improve overall hormonal balance in women over 30.

Maintaining a healthy gut is also crucial for managing weight and digestion, as well as reducing inflammation in the body. When our gut is inflamed, it can lead to a cascade of hormonal imbalances that can impact our weight, digestion, and overall health. By focusing on improving gut health through probiotics and a healthy diet, women over 30 can support their hormonal balance and reduce inflammation in the body.

In conclusion, the gut-hormone connection is a complex and important aspect of women's health, particularly for those over 30. By understanding how our gut health impacts our hormonal balance, we can make informed choices to support our bodies and improve our overall well-being. Incorporating probiotics into our diet is a simple and effective way to promote a healthy gut microbiome, support hormonal balance, and reduce inflammation in the body. By taking care of our gut health, we can empower ourselves to live our best lives and thrive as women over 30.

Supporting Hormonal Balance with Probiotics

As women age, hormonal imbalances can become a common issue that affects overall health and well-being. One way to support hormonal balance is through the use of probiotics, which are beneficial bacteria that promote a healthy gut microbiome. By incorporating probiotics into your daily routine, you can help regulate hormone levels and improve overall gut health.

Probiotics play a key role in supporting hormonal balance by promoting the growth of good bacteria in the gut. These good bacteria help to metabolize and eliminate excess hormones, such as estrogen, which can become imbalanced and lead to symptoms like PMS, mood swings, and weight gain. By maintaining a healthy balance of gut bacteria with probiotics, women over 30 can support their hormonal health and reduce the risk of hormonal imbalances.

In addition to supporting hormonal balance, probiotics can also help with weight management. Imbalances in gut bacteria have been linked to weight gain and obesity, so incorporating probiotics into your diet can help to regulate metabolism and promote a healthy weight. By improving gut health with probiotics, women over 30 can support their weight management goals and maintain a healthy body composition.

Furthermore, probiotics can aid in digestion and reduce inflammation in the gut. Digestive issues like bloating, gas, and constipation can be common as women age, but probiotics can help to improve gut motility and reduce inflammation in the digestive tract. By supporting gut health with probiotics, women over 30 can experience better digestion and reduced inflammation, leading to improved overall health and well-being.

Overall, incorporating probiotics into your daily routine can have a positive impact on hormonal balance, weight management, digestion, and inflammation. By supporting gut health with probiotics, women over 30 can improve their overall health and well-being, leading to a happier and healthier life. Whether you are looking to balance hormones, manage weight, improve digestion, or reduce inflammation, probiotics can be a valuable tool in achieving optimal gut health.

Chapter 6: Incorporating Probiotics into Your Daily Routine

Choosing the Right Probiotic Supplements

Choosing the right probiotic supplements can be overwhelming with so many options on the market today. As women over 30, it is important to prioritize your gut health, as it plays a crucial role in various aspects of your overall well-being, including digestion, weight management, inflammation, and hormonal balance. In this subchapter, we will discuss how to select the best probiotic supplements tailored to your specific needs and goals.

When choosing a probiotic supplement, it is essential to consider the specific strains of bacteria included in the product. Different probiotic strains have varying benefits, so it is crucial to choose a supplement that contains strains that target your specific health concerns. For example, Lactobacillus and Bifidobacterium strains are beneficial for overall gut health and digestion, while certain strains like Lactobacillus rhamnosus may help reduce inflammation in the gut.

In addition to considering the strains of bacteria, it is important to look for a probiotic supplement that contains a high number of colony-forming units (CFUs). CFUs indicate the amount of live bacteria in the supplement, which is crucial for ensuring its efficacy. As a general rule of thumb, look for probiotic supplements that contain at least 10 billion CFUs per serving to ensure you are getting an adequate dose of beneficial bacteria.

It is also essential to choose a probiotic supplement that is backed by scientific research and has been tested for safety and efficacy. Look for products that have undergone third-party testing and have certifications from reputable organizations to ensure that you are getting a high-quality supplement. Reading reviews from other women over 30 who have tried the product can also provide valuable insights into its effectiveness.

Lastly, it is important to consult with a healthcare provider or a registered dietitian before starting any new supplement regimen, especially if you have underlying health conditions or are taking medications. They can help you determine the best probiotic supplement for your individual needs and provide guidance on how to integrate it into your daily routine for optimal results. By choosing the right probiotic supplement tailored to your specific needs, you can support your gut health and overall well-being as a woman over 30.

Adding Probiotic-Rich Foods to Your Diet

As women over 30, it's important to prioritize our gut health in order to maintain overall wellness. One way to support our digestive system is by incorporating probiotic-rich foods into our diet. Probiotics are live bacteria and yeasts that are beneficial for our gut health, helping to balance the microbiome and support proper digestion.

Probiotics for gut health are essential for maintaining a healthy balance of bacteria in the gut. By adding probiotic-rich foods such as yogurt, kefir, sauerkraut, and kimchi to our diet, we can introduce beneficial bacteria that help to improve digestion and reduce inflammation in the gut. These foods can also help to support our immune system and protect against harmful bacteria that can lead to digestive issues.

Incorporating probiotic-rich foods into our diet can also aid in weight management. Research has shown that a healthy gut microbiome is essential for maintaining a healthy weight, as imbalances in gut bacteria have been linked to obesity and weight gain. By consuming probiotic-rich foods regularly, we can help to support a healthy balance of bacteria in the gut and improve our body's ability to metabolize food efficiently.

Additionally, probiotics can help to support hormonal balance in women over 30. Our gut health plays a crucial role in hormone regulation, as imbalances in gut bacteria can lead to hormonal disruptions that can impact our mood, energy levels, and overall well-being. By incorporating probiotic-rich foods into our diet, we can help to support a healthy balance of hormones and improve our overall hormonal health.

In conclusion, adding probiotic-rich foods to our diet is essential for women over 30 looking to support their gut health, aid in weight management, improve digestion, reduce inflammation, and support hormonal balance. By incorporating foods such as yogurt, kefir, sauerkraut, and kimchi into our daily meals, we can introduce beneficial bacteria that will help to improve our overall wellness and support a healthy gut microbiome. Remember, a healthy gut is the foundation for overall well-being, so prioritize your digestive health by adding probiotic-rich foods to your diet today.

Chapter 7: Maintaining Gut Health for Long-Term Wellness

Lifestyle Factors That Impact Gut Health

In this subchapter, we will explore the lifestyle factors that can have a significant impact on your gut health. As women over 30, it is essential to understand how various aspects of our daily routines can either support or hinder the health of our digestive system. By making small changes in our lifestyle, we can improve our gut health and overall well-being.

One of the most critical lifestyle factors that influence gut health is diet. Consuming a balanced diet rich in fiber, fruits, vegetables, and whole grains is essential for maintaining a healthy gut microbiome. Probiotic-rich foods such as yogurt, kefir, and sauerkraut can also help promote the growth of beneficial bacteria in the gut. On the other hand, a diet high in processed foods, sugar, and unhealthy fats can disrupt the balance of gut bacteria and lead to digestive issues.

In addition to diet, stress management plays a crucial role in gut health. Chronic stress can negatively impact the gut microbiome and contribute to digestive problems such as bloating, gas, and constipation. Finding ways to reduce stress, such as practicing mindfulness, meditation, yoga, or deep breathing exercises, can help support a healthy gut.

Regular physical activity is another lifestyle factor that can influence gut health. Exercise has been shown to have a positive impact on gut microbiota composition and diversity. Aim to incorporate a mix of cardiovascular, strength training, and flexibility exercises into your routine to support a healthy gut and overall wellness.

Getting an adequate amount of sleep is also essential for gut health. Poor sleep habits can disrupt the balance of gut bacteria and lead to digestive issues. Aim for 7-9 hours of quality sleep each night to support a healthy gut microbiome. By making small changes to your diet, stress management, physical activity, and sleep habits, you can improve your gut health and overall well-being as a woman over 30.

Creating a Gut-Healthy Plan for Women Over 30

As women age, maintaining gut health becomes increasingly important for overall wellness. In your 30s and beyond, the gut microbiome can become imbalanced due to factors such as stress, poor diet, and hormonal changes. Creating a gut-healthy plan tailored specifically for women over 30 can help support digestive wellness, weight management, hormonal balance, and reduce inflammation.

Probiotics are key players in promoting gut health for women over 30. These beneficial bacteria help maintain a balanced gut microbiome, which is essential for proper digestion and overall health. Incorporating probiotic-rich foods such as yogurt, kefir, sauerkraut, and kimchi into your diet can help support a healthy gut flora. Additionally, taking a high-quality probiotic supplement can further support gut health and promote optimal digestion.

Weight management can be a challenge for many women over 30, but a gut-healthy plan can help support a healthy weight. Research has shown that an imbalanced gut microbiome can contribute to weight gain and obesity. By focusing on gut health through probiotics and a nutrient-dense diet, women can support their metabolism and promote weight loss. Additionally, incorporating regular exercise and stress management techniques can further support weight management goals.

Digestive issues such as bloating, constipation, and indigestion can be common concerns for women over 30. A gut-healthy plan can help alleviate these symptoms and promote optimal digestion. By including fiber-rich foods, such as fruits, vegetables, and whole grains, in your diet, you can support healthy digestion and prevent constipation. Additionally, staying hydrated and practicing mindful eating can further support digestive wellness.

Inflammation is a common issue that can contribute to a variety of health problems, including digestive issues, hormonal imbalances, and weight gain. A gut-healthy plan for women over 30 can help reduce inflammation and promote overall wellness. Including anti-inflammatory foods such as fatty fish, nuts, seeds, and leafy greens in your diet can help combat inflammation and support gut health. Additionally, avoiding processed foods, sugar, and trans fats can further reduce inflammation in the body.

Hormonal balance is essential for women over 30, as imbalances can contribute to a variety of health issues, including digestive problems. A gut-healthy plan can help support hormonal balance and promote overall wellness. By focusing on gut health through probiotics and a balanced diet, women can support hormone production and regulation. Additionally, incorporating stress management techniques such as yoga, meditation, and deep breathing exercises can further support hormonal balance and overall well-being. By creating a gut-healthy plan tailored specifically for women over 30, you can support digestive wellness, weight management, hormonal balance, and reduce inflammation for optimal health and vitality.

Chapter 8: Tracking Your Progress and Making Adjustments

Monitoring Gut Health Changes

As women over 30, it is important to pay close attention to our gut health in order to maintain overall well-being. One way to do this is by monitoring any changes in our gut health. Keeping track of how our digestive system is functioning can help us identify potential issues early on and take steps to address them before they become more serious.

One way to monitor gut health changes is by paying attention to our digestion. If you notice changes in your bowel movements, such as constipation, diarrhea, or irregularity, it could be a sign that something is off with your gut health. Keeping a food diary can help you identify any triggers that may be causing digestive issues and allow you to make necessary adjustments to your diet.

Another important aspect of monitoring gut health changes is paying attention to any symptoms of inflammation. Inflammation in the gut can lead to a host of health issues, including bloating, gas, and discomfort. If you notice any of these symptoms, it may be a sign that your gut health is not optimal. Incorporating probiotics into your diet can help reduce inflammation and promote a healthy gut environment.

Weight management is also closely linked to gut health, so monitoring any changes in your weight can provide valuable insight into the state of your digestive system. Sudden weight gain or loss could be a sign of gut health issues, such as an imbalance of good and bad bacteria in the gut. By maintaining a healthy weight through proper diet and exercise, you can support your gut health and overall well-being.

Lastly, hormonal balance plays a key role in gut health for women over 30. Fluctuations in hormones can impact the gut microbiome and lead to digestive issues. Keeping track of any changes in your menstrual cycle, mood swings, or skin health can provide clues about your hormonal balance and its effect on your gut health. By addressing hormonal imbalances through lifestyle changes and possibly seeking medical advice, you can support your gut health and promote overall wellness. Monitoring gut health changes is essential for women over 30 to maintain optimal digestive wellness and overall well-being. By paying attention to digestion, inflammation, weight management, and hormonal balance, you can take proactive steps to support your gut health and address any issues that may arise. Incorporating probiotics into your diet, maintaining a healthy weight, and balancing hormones can all contribute to a healthy gut environment and promote digestive wellness. Remember to listen to your body and seek medical advice if you notice any concerning changes in your gut health. Your gut health is a key component of your overall well-being, so it is important to prioritize monitoring and maintaining it for a healthier and happier life.

Adjusting Probiotic Intake as Needed

In order to optimize the benefits of probiotics for gut health, it's important to adjust your intake as needed. As women over 30, our bodies are constantly changing and our gut health needs may vary depending on various factors such as stress levels, diet, and overall health. By being mindful of these factors, we can tailor our probiotic intake to meet our individual needs.

One way to adjust probiotic intake is to pay attention to how your body responds to different strains and dosages. Some women may find that they need a higher dosage of probiotics to maintain gut health, while others may do well with a lower dosage. By experimenting with different probiotic supplements and observing how your body reacts, you can determine the right balance for your unique needs.

Another factor to consider when adjusting probiotic intake is the quality of the probiotic supplements you are taking. Not all probiotics are created equal, and some may be more effective than others in promoting gut health. Look for supplements that contain a variety of strains, as diversity in your gut microbiome is key to overall digestive wellness.

It's also important to listen to your body and make adjustments to your probiotic intake as needed. If you are experiencing digestive issues such as bloating, gas, or irregular bowel movements, it may be a sign that you need to increase or decrease your probiotic intake. Consulting with a healthcare provider or a registered dietitian can help you make informed decisions about adjusting your probiotic regimen.

In conclusion, adjusting probiotic intake as needed is essential for maintaining optimal gut health as women over 30. By paying attention to how your body responds to different strains and dosages, choosing high-quality supplements, and listening to your body's signals, you can tailor your probiotic intake to support digestion, weight management, inflammation, and hormonal balance. Remember, every woman is unique, so it's important to find the right balance that works best for you.

Chapter 9: Additional Resources for Women Over 30

Recommended Books and Websites

In this subchapter, we will explore some recommended books and websites that can provide valuable information and guidance for women over 30 looking to improve their gut health through probiotics. These resources cover a range of topics related to gut health, including weight management, digestion, inflammation, and hormonal balance.

One highly recommended book for women interested in probiotics for gut health is "The Microbiome Solution" by Dr. Robynne Chutkan. This book offers practical advice on how to cultivate a healthy gut microbiome through diet, lifestyle changes, and the use of probiotic supplements. Dr. Chutkan's approach is science-based and easy to understand, making it a valuable resource for women looking to improve their digestive wellness.

For women interested in the connection between gut health and weight management, "The Good Gut Diet" by Gerard Mullin is a must-read. This book provides a comprehensive guide to using probiotics to support weight loss and maintain a healthy body composition. Mullin's research-backed recommendations can help women over 30 achieve their weight loss goals while also improving their gut health.

Another valuable resource for women seeking to improve their gut health and digestion is the website Healthline.com. This website offers a wealth of information on probiotics, digestive health, and gut-friendly recipes. Healthline's articles are written by medical professionals and nutrition experts, making it a reliable source of information for women looking to optimize their digestive wellness.

Women interested in the role of gut health in inflammation may find "The Inflammation Spectrum" by Dr. Will Cole to be a valuable resource. This book explores the connection between gut health and chronic inflammation, offering practical advice on how to reduce inflammation through diet, lifestyle changes, and targeted supplements. Dr. Cole's holistic approach to inflammation can help women over 30 manage inflammatory conditions and improve their overall health.

For women looking to balance their hormones through gut health, the website HormoneBalanceNutrition.com is a valuable resource. This website offers evidence-based information on how gut health influences hormonal balance, as well as practical tips for supporting hormone health through probiotics and other gut-friendly strategies. Women over 30 seeking to optimize their hormonal health can benefit from the expert advice and resources available on HormoneBalanceNutrition.com.

Support Groups and Communities for Gut Health

Support groups and communities can be invaluable resources for women over 30 looking to improve their gut health. These groups provide a sense of community and camaraderie, as well as a space to share experiences and tips for managing digestive issues. Whether you are looking to learn more about probiotics for gut health, explore the connection between gut health and weight management, or seeking advice on how to improve digestion, joining a support group can provide you with the knowledge and support you need to make positive changes in your life.

One of the key benefits of joining a support group for gut health is the opportunity to learn from others who have similar experiences. By sharing your own struggles and successes, you can gain valuable insights and advice from women who have been through similar challenges. This sense of community can be empowering and motivating, helping you to stay on track with your gut health goals. Additionally, support groups often provide access to expert advice and resources, giving you the tools you need to make informed decisions about your health.

For women over 30 interested in probiotics for gut health, support groups can be a great way to learn more about the benefits of these beneficial bacteria. Probiotics have been shown to support digestive health, boost the immune system, and even improve mental health. By connecting with others who are knowledgeable about probiotics, you can gain a deeper understanding of how these supplements can benefit your gut health and overall well-being. Support groups may also provide recommendations for specific probiotic strains and products that have been effective for other members.

Gut health and weight management are closely linked, and joining a support group can help you navigate this complex relationship. Women over 30 often struggle with maintaining a healthy weight as they age, and gut health plays a crucial role in metabolism and digestion. By connecting with others who are also working towards weight management goals, you can share tips and strategies for improving gut health and reaching your ideal weight. Support groups may offer guidance on incorporating gut-friendly foods into your diet, as well as tips for managing cravings and emotional eating.

Inflammation, hormonal balance, and digestion are all key components of gut health, and support groups can provide valuable insights into how to optimize these areas of your health. By connecting with other women who are also interested in improving their gut health, you can gain new perspectives on how to reduce inflammation, balance hormones, and support healthy digestion. Support groups may offer resources such as meal plans, recipes, and lifestyle tips that can help you make positive changes in these areas. Overall, joining a support group focused on gut health can provide you with the knowledge, encouragement, and motivation you need to take control of your digestive wellness and improve your overall health and well-being.

Chapter 10: Conclusion

Recap of Key Points

In this subchapter, we will recap some key points discussed in this book "Probiotics and Gut Health: A Woman's Guide to Digestive Wellness," specifically tailored to women over 30 who are interested in improving their gut health and overall wellbeing. Throughout this book, we have explored the importance of probiotics for gut health and how they can positively impact digestion, weight management, inflammation, and hormonal balance in women.

One of the key points to remember is that probiotics are beneficial bacteria that can help maintain a healthy balance in the gut microbiome. These good bacteria can aid in digestion, reduce inflammation, and support overall gut health. It is important for women over 30 to incorporate probiotic-rich foods such as yogurt, kefir, sauerkraut, and kimchi into their diets to promote a diverse and healthy gut microbiome.

Another important point to consider is the connection between gut health and weight management. Research has shown that an imbalance in the gut microbiome can contribute to weight gain and obesity. By incorporating probiotics into your diet, you can support a healthy gut microbiome and potentially aid in weight management. Additionally, probiotics may help regulate hormones that influence metabolism and appetite, further supporting weight management efforts.

Furthermore, gut health plays a crucial role in digestion and nutrient absorption. A healthy gut microbiome can help break down food, absorb essential nutrients, and promote regular bowel movements. By maintaining a diverse and balanced gut microbiome through probiotic-rich foods and supplements, women over 30 can support optimal digestion and nutrient absorption.

In addition to digestion and weight management, gut health also plays a role in inflammation and hormonal balance in women. An imbalance in the gut microbiome can lead to chronic inflammation, which has been linked to various health conditions such as autoimmune disorders, heart disease, and obesity. By supporting a healthy gut microbiome with probiotics, women over 30 can potentially reduce inflammation and promote overall wellbeing.

In conclusion, maintaining a healthy gut microbiome through probiotics is essential for women over 30 who are looking to improve their digestive wellness. By incorporating probiotic-rich foods and supplements into your diet, you can support digestion, weight management, inflammation, and hormonal balance. Remember to prioritize your gut health and make informed choices that promote a diverse and balanced gut microbiome for optimal wellbeing.

Committing to Gut Health for a Vibrant Life

As women over 30, we know how important it is to take care of our bodies in order to live a vibrant and fulfilling life. One key aspect of overall health that often gets overlooked is gut health. Our gut is home to trillions of bacteria that play a crucial role in our digestion, immunity, and overall well-being. By committing to gut health, we can experience numerous benefits that will enhance our quality of life.

Probiotics are a powerful tool in the quest for optimal gut health. These beneficial bacteria help to maintain a healthy balance in our gut microbiome, which is essential for proper digestion and immunity. By incorporating probiotic-rich foods like yogurt, kefir, and sauerkraut into our diets, we can support the growth of good bacteria in our guts and improve our overall health. Probiotic supplements are also available for those who may need an extra boost in maintaining a healthy gut flora.

Maintaining a healthy gut is also essential for weight management. Research has shown that the balance of bacteria in our gut can influence our metabolism and the way our bodies store fat. By promoting the growth of good bacteria through probiotics and fiber-rich foods, we can support a healthy weight and reduce the risk of obesity. When our gut is healthy, we are better able to absorb nutrients from our food and maintain a balanced weight.

In addition to weight management, gut health is also closely linked to digestion. When our gut is out of balance, we may experience symptoms like bloating, gas, and constipation. By focusing on gut-friendly foods like fiber-rich vegetables, whole grains, and fermented foods, we can support a healthy digestive system and reduce these uncomfortable symptoms. Probiotics can also help to improve digestion by promoting the growth of beneficial bacteria that aid in the breakdown of food.

Furthermore, maintaining a healthy gut can also help to reduce inflammation in the body. Chronic inflammation has been linked to a number of health issues, including heart disease, arthritis, and autoimmune disorders. By supporting our gut health with probiotics and anti-inflammatory foods like fatty fish, berries, and leafy greens, we can help to reduce overall inflammation in the body and protect ourselves from these serious health conditions. A healthy gut is the foundation for a healthy body, and by committing to gut health, we can experience lasting benefits for our overall well-being.

Lastly, gut health is closely tied to hormonal balance in women. The gut microbiome plays a key role in metabolizing hormones like estrogen and progesterone, and an imbalance in gut bacteria can lead to hormonal issues like PMS, irregular periods, and menopausal symptoms. By nourishing our gut with probiotics and hormone-balancing foods like flaxseeds, cruciferous vegetables, and green tea, we can support a healthy balance of hormones and reduce the symptoms of hormonal imbalances. Taking care of our gut health is essential for supporting our hormonal balance and overall well-being as women over 30.